The

Eat Less Crap

And

Get Off Your Arse

Diet

Stefano V Verde

Stefano V Verde

Stefano V Verde is not a Doctor, or a qualified Dietitian. However, he is an observer of Human behaviour. After studying people with weight issues for many years, Stefano has developed his revolutionary diet - a diet so simple - that it is just amazing.

DEDICATION

FOR DAD

ACKNOWLEDGMENTS

The inspiration for the diet, and this book, came from a workmate of mine. He had noticed that I'd put on a little weight. Being a sensitive soul he said "Stefano, the only thing stopping you from going to Weight Watchers is the door frame - yer fat bastard"

WARNING!

You need to read the forward before starting this book.

Forward:

Your journey to slimmer healthier you starts here. You will be amazed just how simple it is. You will need a bookmark (or the ability to fold down the corner of a page) and a drop of willpower.

All you have to do is keep this book by your bed and read one page each morning. Follow the instructions on that page, and you should start to see results in no time.

Don't forget to check the Glossary on page 31 for my definition of "Crap" and "Off Your Arse"

p.s Always consult with your doctor before starting a new diet or fitness program.

<u>DAY 1</u>

Eat Less Crap

(See Glossary for definition of "Crap")

And

Get Off Your

Arse!

(See Glossary for definition of "getting off your arse")

Read the next page tomorrow

Good Luck!

Weight:

Fitness: POOR FAIR GOOD

(Circle one)

<u>DAY 2</u>

Eat Less Crap

And

Get Off Your

Arse!

Read the next page tomorrow

Good Luck!

Weight:

Fitness: POOR FAIR GOOD

(Circle one)

DAY 3

Eat Less Crap

And

Get Off Your

Arse!

Read the next page tomorrow

Good Luck!

Weight:

Fitness: POOR FAIR GOOD

(Circle one)

DAY 4

Eat Less Crap

And

Get Off Your

Arse!

Read the next page tomorrow

Good Luck!

Weight:

Fitness: POOR FAIR GOOD

(Circle one)

DAY 5

Eat Less Crap

And

Get Off Your

Arse!

Read the next page tomorrow

Good Luck!

Weight:

Fitness: POOR FAIR GOOD

(Circle one)

DAY 6

Eat Less Crap

And

Get Off Your

Arse!

Read the next page tomorrow

Good Luck!

Weight:

Fitness: POOR FAIR GOOD

(Circle one)

DAY 7

Eat Less Crap

And

Get Off Your

Arse!

Read the next page tomorrow

Good Luck!

Weight:

Fitness: POOR FAIR GOOD

(Circle one)

DAY 8

Eat Less Crap

And

Get Off Your

Arse!

Read the next page tomorrow

Good Luck!

Weight:

Fitness: POOR FAIR GOOD

(Circle one)

<u>DAY 9</u>

Eat Less Crap

And

Get Off Your

Arse!

Read the next page tomorrow

Good Luck!

Weight:

Fitness: POOR FAIR GOOD

(Circle one)

<u>DAY 10</u>

Eat Less Crap

And

Get Off Your

Arse!

Read the next page tomorrow

Good Luck!

Weight:

Fitness: POOR FAIR GOOD

(Circle one)

<u>DAY 11</u>

Eat Less Crap

And

Get Off Your

Arse!

Read the next page tomorrow

Good Luck!

Weight:

Fitness: POOR FAIR GOOD

(Circle one)

DAY 12

Eat Less Crap

And

Get Off Your

Arse!

Read the next page tomorrow

Good Luck!

Weight:

Fitness: POOR FAIR GOOD

(Circle one)

<u>DAY 13</u>

Eat Less Crap

And

Get Off Your

Arse!

Read the next page tomorrow

Good Luck!

Weight:

Fitness: POOR FAIR GOOD

(Circle one)

DAY 14

Eat Less Crap

And

Get Off Your

Arse!

Read the next page tomorrow

Good Luck!

Weight:

Fitness: POOR FAIR GOOD

(Circle one)

STEFANO V VERDE

Congratulations!

You've completed the first two weeks of the "Eat Less Crap And Get Off Your Arse Diet"

If you have followed the instructions carefully, you should now weigh less and feel healthier.

Also, you should have a good grasp of the finer detail of this diet plan (If not, go back to page one).

What now? Can you guess? You've got it:

Eat Less Crap

And

Get Off Your

Arse!

For the rest of your longer, healthier life.

Glossary of terms:

Crap: Crisps (chips U.S), Biscuits, cookies, cakes, sweets (candy U.S), doughnuts, muffins, puddings, desserts - I think you get the picture - stuff we eat and drink that is generally seen as a snack, or an extra part of a meal. This may surprise you, but I do not consider foods such as burgers, hot dogs and pizza as crap. They are foods, but they are foods that should be eaten once or twice a week, not once or twice a day.

Most foods are good for us, it's just the frequency and quantity that we eat them that can make them good or bad for our health. Eating what we call "good" foods in quantities large enough to make a pig sick will have a negative effect on our health.

It is a fact that you can eat three filling and healthy meals a day without going over your recommended daily calorie intake - you just have to cut out all the other crap. As a rule, people do not get fat because of their: Genes/Glands/Race/Gender/Shoes or Shampoo. People get fat because of the amount they eat and how little they do.

Glossary of terms (Cont'd):

Getting off your arse: This part is simple: to lose weight you must burn off more calories than you eat. That does not mean eat to few calories for your gender/build. It means that if you're eating the recommended number of calories (1940 calories per day for women and 2550 for men), then you must exercise if you want to lose weight. A manual worker who takes in the recommended number of calories will tend to be lean. An office worker (who doesn't exercise) doing the same will tend to be flabby, but you already knew that.

I am not talking about a massive amount of exercise. Just enough to get you a bit of a sweat on. Half an hour of brisk walking each day - combined with a crap free diet - and you should see the needle on the scales heading in the right direction, but you already knew that. Obviously, the more you get off your arse, the faster you will shift the pounds.

Now, did you really need me to tell you this? I thought not. You know what to do - you always have - Eat less crap and get off your arse.

Good Luck!

Stefano V Verde

END

ABOUT THE AUTHOR

Stefano is a former Royal Naval Engineer. After 16 years service, spent mostly eating, drinking and smoking too much, he decided enough was enough. With the scales hitting 16 stone (224 pounds), Stefano developed a Diet system that was both revolutionary and simple. The rest, as they say, is history......

www.ingramcontent.com/pod-product-compliance
Lightning Source LLC
Chambersburg PA
CBHW070237290526
45789CB00004B/1668